WORK SMART NOT HARD

Lazy Ways To Transform Your Body And Mind

By

HARLEY MIDDLETON

TABLE OF CONTENTS

SECTION I

THE POWER OF LAZINESS

Effortless Eating:Focus on whole, minimally processed foods. Keep healthy snacks like fruits, nuts, or cut veggies readily available. This lazy approach reduces the temptation to indulge in less nutritious options.

Lazy Workouts that Work:Opt for short, intense exercises like 20-minute HIIT sessions. These burn calories effectively, making your workout efficient and leaving more time for relaxation.

Snooze to Lose: Prioritize 7-9 hours of quality sleep each night. This lazy yet essential habit helps regulate hunger hormones (ghrelin and leptin), making it easier to resist unhealthy food cravings.

Fun Fitness: Choose activities you genuinely enjoy. Whether it's dancing, cycling, or playing a favorite sport, incorporating enjoyable activities makes staying active feel like a leisurely pursuit rather than a strenuous effort.

Hydration Habit: Keep a water bottle nearby. Lazily sipping water throughout the day not only supports metabolism but also helps control appetite, making it easier to resist the urge to snack on less healthy options.

CAN WEIGHT LOSS LOWER BLOOD PRESSURE

Yes, weight loss can often lead to a reduction in blood pressure. When you lose weight, especially if it involves a reduction in body fat, it can positively impact various factors related to blood pressure:

Reduced Volume of Blood: Losing weight can decrease the amount of blood your heart needs to pump, resulting in lower blood pressure.

Improved Cardiovascular Health:Weight loss is often associated with improvements in cardiovascular health, including better function of the heart and blood vessels.

Decreased Resistance in Arteries:Excess weight can contribute to increased resistance in the arteries, leading to higher blood pressure. Losing weight can help reduce this resistance.

Balanced Hormones:Weight loss can lead to better hormone balance, particularly in insulin sensitivity. This can positively influence blood pressure regulation.

However, individual responses vary, and other factors such as genetics, diet, physical activity, and stress also play a role in blood pressure regulation. It's essential to approach weight loss as part of an overall healthy lifestyle, including a balanced diet and regular physical activity, for the most sustainable benefits. If you have concerns about your blood pressure or weight, it's advisable to consult with a healthcare professional.

INVOLUNTARY WEIGHT REDUCTION

Losing weight without actively trying often involves making subtle lifestyle changes. Here are some tips:

Mindful Eating: Pay attention to what you eat. Listen to your body's hunger and fullness cues, and avoid distractions while eating.

Portion Control:Be mindful of portion sizes. Using smaller plates can help control the amount of food you consume without feeling like you're restricting yourself.

Choose Nutrient-Dense Foods:Opt for foods that are rich in nutrients but lower in calories. This includes fruits, vegetables, lean proteins, and whole grains.

Stay Hydrated:Drinking water before meals can help you feel fuller, potentially reducing the amount of food you eat.

Regular Physical Activity:Incorporate gentle, regular physical activity into your routine, such as walking or taking the stairs. It can contribute to weight maintenance without intense effort.

Remember, sustainable weight loss often involves gradual changes over time. If you have specific health concerns or goals, it's advisable to consult with a healthcare professional or a registered dietitian for personalized advice.

SECTION II

AS A WOMAN, HOW CAN I LOSE WEIGHT?

"Making a few simple life changes can help promote long-lasting weight loss for women. Doing just 1 or 2 of these each day can help maximize results and promote healthy, sustainable weight loss. Diet and exercise may be key components of weight loss for women, but many other factors play a role.

In fact, studies show that everything from sleep quality to stress levels can have a major impact on hunger, metabolism, body weight, and belly fat.

Fortunately, making a few small changes in your daily routine can bring big benefits when it comes to weight loss.

Cut Down On Refined Carbs:Refined carbs undergo extensive processing, reducing the amount of fiber and micronutrients in the final product. These foods spike blood sugar levels, increase hunger, and are associated with increased body weight and belly fat. Therefore, it's best to limit refined carbs like white bread, pasta, and prepackaged foods. Opt for whole-grain products like oats, brown rice, quinoa, buckwheat, and barley instead.

Add Resistance Training to Your Routine: Resistance training builds muscle and increases endurance. It's especially beneficial for women over 50, as it increases the number of calories your body burns at rest. It also helps preserve bone mineral density to protect against osteoporosis. Lifting weights, using gym equipment, or performing body-weight exercises are a few simple ways to get started.

Drink More Water: Drinking more water is an easy and effective way to promote weight loss with minimal effort. According to one small study, drinking 16.9 ounces (500 ml) of water temporarily increased the number of calories burned by 30% after 30–40 minutes.

Set a Regular Sleep Schedule: Studies suggest that getting enough sleep may be just as crucial to losing weight as diet and exercise. Multiple studies have associated sleep deprivation with increased body weight and higher levels of ghrelin, the hormone responsible for stimulating hunger. Furthermore, one study in women showed that getting at least seven hours of sleep each night and improving overall sleep quality increased the likelihood of weight loss success by 33%

Keep a Food Journal: Using a food journal to track what you eat is an easy way to hold yourself accountable and make healthier choices. It also makes it easier to count calories, which can be an effective strategy for weight management. What's more, a food journal can help you stick to your goals and may result in greater long-term weight loss."

NATURAL WAYS FOR MEN TO ACHIEVE WEIGHT LOSS

Balanced Diet:

What They Need: A diet rich in whole foods – fruits, vegetables, lean proteins, and whole grains. Adequate protein intake is essential for muscle maintenance and weight loss. How It Helps: Provides necessary nutrients, controls hunger, and supports metabolism

Regular Exercise:

What They Need: A combination of strength training and cardiovascular exercise.

How It Helps: Builds muscle, burns calories, and improves overall fitness. Strength training helps maintain muscle mass, crucial for weight loss.

Adequate Hydration:

What They Need: Plenty of water throughout the day.

How It Helps:Helps control appetite, supports metabolism, and ensures proper bodily functions.

Quality Sleep:

What They Need:7-9 hours of uninterrupted sleep

How It Helps: Regulates hormones related to hunger and stress, supporting weight loss

Mindful Eating:

What They Need: Awareness of portion sizes and eating without distractions.

How It Helps: Promotes healthier food choices and prevents overeating.

Limit Refined Carbs and Sugars:

What They Need: Reduction in processed foods, sugary drinks, and white bread.

How It Helps: Controls blood sugar levels, reduces cravings, and supports weight loss.

Stress Management:

What They Need: Techniques like meditation, deep breathing, or engaging in hobbies.

How It Helps: Manages stress hormones that can contribute to weight gain.

Consistent Routine:

What They Need: A consistent schedule for meals, exercise, and sleep.

How It Helps: Establishes healthy habits and supports weight loss efforts.

Fiber-Rich Foods:

What They Need:High-fiber foods like fruits, vegetables, and whole grains.

How It Helps: Enhances satiety, supports digestion, and aids in weight management.

Social Support:

What They Need:Encouragement from friends, family, or a support group.

How It Helps:Provides motivation, accountability, and emotional support.

By incorporating these natural approaches into their lifestyle, men can achieve sustainable and healthy weight loss. Remember, consistency is key, and gradual changes lead to long-term success.

SECTION III

STRENGTH AND CARDIOVASCULAR FITNESS

Strength:

Building strength involves working your muscles against resistance. This can be through activities like weightlifting, bodyweight exercises (like squats and push-ups), or using resistance bands. The benefits of strength training include:

Increased muscle mass: Makes daily activities easier.

Improved metabolism: Helps burn more calories even at rest.

• Better bone health: Strength training can enhance bone density.

• Enhanced joint function: Strength training supports joint health.

Cardiovascular Fitness:

Cardio fitness focuses on improving the health of your heart and lungs. Activities like brisk walking, running, cycling, or dancing get your heart rate up. The perks of cardiovascular fitness include:

• Improved heart health: Strengthens your heart muscle.

• Enhanced lung capacity: Improves the efficiency of oxygen intake.

• Weight management: Burns calories and supports weight loss.

- Stress reduction: Cardio exercises release endorphins, reducing stress.

Why Combine Both:

Comprehensive Fitness:Strength and cardio together provide a well-rounded fitness routine.

Heart Health:Cardiovascular exercise complements strength training by promoting a healthy heart.

Weight Management:The combo helps burn calories, aiding in weight loss or maintenance.

Energy Boost: Improved stamina from cardio and strength enhances overall energy levels.

Versatility: You can tailor your routine to include activities you enjoy, making fitness more sustainable.

So, whether it's lifting weights or going for a run, incorporating both strength and cardiovascular exercises into your routine is like giving your body the ultimate fitness experience.

HOW BRAIN AND NEURO UPGRADES WORK

Savor Every Bite: Train your brain to enjoy and appreciate each mouthful.Naturally prevents overeating as your brain becomes better at recognizing when you're satisfied.

Visualize Your Success: Picture yourself reaching your weight loss goals regularly.Boosts motivation without extra effort, making healthier choices feel more instinctive.

Enjoyable Exercise Routine: Find exercises you genuinely like. Makes working out a more enjoyable part of your routine, reducing the need for sheer willpower.

Reward Small Wins: Treat yourself for achieving small milestones. Creates a sense of accomplishment that naturally encourages ongoing progress.

Stress-Busting Techniques: Use stress-reduction practices like meditation.Lowers stress-induced cravings and emotional eating, making weight loss feel less challenging.

Change Cravings Patterns: Swap out unhealthy triggers with better alternatives. Shifts your brain's signals toward healthier food choices effortlessly.

Prioritize Restful Sleep: Make quality sleep a priority.Supports weight loss by regulating hunger hormones, no extra effort required.

Surround Yourself with Positivity: Seek supportive influences.Creates a natural environment that reinforces healthier choices.

Associate Water with Refreshment: Link drinking water to feeling revitalized.Encourages regular hydration without needing to constantly remind yourself.

Make Habits Stick: Repeat healthy actions consistently.

Turns positive behaviors into automatic habits for sustained, 'lazy' weight loss success.

By training your brain with these simple but powerful upgrades, weight loss becomes more intuitive, making a healthier lifestyle feel like second nature."

THE POWER OF EVALUATE, PERSONALIZE AND REPEAT

Understandable Explanation: Take a look at your daily routines and habits.
Identify patterns like snacking or sedentary behaviors. Recognizing what you're currently doing is the first step to making positive changes.

Personalize Your Approach: Tailor your plan to fit your preferences and lifestyle.

Choose exercises you enjoy and foods that suit your taste. Personalizing your approach makes it more likely that you'll stick with it for the long haul.

Repeat What Works: Stick to the strategies that bring you success.

If morning workouts are effective for you, keep doing them. Repeating successful actions creates consistency, making your healthy choices more automatic.

How This Helps with Weight Loss: Look at what you're currently doing.

Assess your eating habits, exercise routine, and sleep patterns. Understanding your starting point helps you set realistic goals.

Personalize: Make your plan suit you.

If you're not a fan of running, find other exercises you enjoy. If you love certain foods, find healthier versions or incorporate them wisely. A personalized plan is more sustainable.

Repeat: Stick to what works well.

If a particular meal prep routine helps you make healthier choices, make it a regular part of your week. Consistency is key to building lasting habits.

By evaluating, personalizing, and repeating successful strategies, you create a weight loss plan that's tailored to you. It's not about one-size-fits-all solutions; it's about finding what works for you and making it a lasting part of your lifestyle.

CONCLUSION

Achieving and maintaining weight loss is a personalized journey that involves understanding, adapting, and consistently applying effective strategies. By evaluating your current habits, personalizing your approach to fit your preferences, and repeating what works for you, you can create a sustainable and enjoyable path towards a healthier lifestyle.

Remember, there is no one-size-fits-all solution, and the key to long-term success lies in making gradual, positive changes that align with your unique needs and preferences. Whether it's through mindful eating, enjoyable exercises, or better sleep habits, finding what works for you and incorporating it into your routine can lead to not only weight loss but also improved overall well-being.

Remember, making small changes over time is the way to go. Celebrate the good stuff, and don't worry if things don't always go perfectly. Keep doing what works for you, and you'll see progress in the long run. So, here's to your success on your weight loss journey – keep going!